GUIDELINES
TO THE USE OF
AGGRESSIVE

COMPASSIONATE
CARE
INSTEAD OF
EUTHANASIA

GUIDELINES TO THE USE OF AGGRESSIVE

COMPASSIONATE CARE INSTEAD OF EUTHANASIA

Dr. F. S. H. Dartana, M. D. LMCC.

Tropical medicine '59-'69. Translation-work since disabled and retired

To order additional copies of this book, contact:
Xlibris Corporation
1-888-795-4274
www.Xlibris.com
Orders@Xlibris.com
55637

TABLE OF CONTENTS

This article on Compassionate Care instead of Euthanasia is tremendous, timely and goal directed. It line by line pulls down the lies and deception that seems to be fueling the Euthanasia drive. Again, the light of God's Word exposes and expels the darkness of the enemy.

PASTOR CAL SWITZER
Victory Christian Center
Edmonton, Alberta, Canada

DEDICATION

I dedicate this booklet to Jesus,
my personal Savior and Lord.
I realize that it is only
a small contribution to His work,
but I hope that it will reach many
who are searching for the truth!

It is unfortunate
that so many kinds of philosophies
are circulating around us.
We are often tempted to pick and choose
what suits us best, especially
in the area of conducting our lives and our deaths.
We like to quote from the Bible
that we have a free will to choose,
which of course is true.
But by choosing, we also choose consequences,
and, of course, we claim to know all about them!

I choose to believe Jesus, Who said:
"I AM the Way, the Truth, and the Life.
No one comes to the Father except through Me."
(John 14:6)

October, 1998

ACKNOWLEDGEMENTS

My very special thanks are given to Pastor Cal Switzer and Father Albert Laisnez for their special encouragements.

I hereby thank Mae Fraser for her excellent help in typing this manuscript for me. I also thank my daughter, Joanne Dartana, who has kindly assisted me in corrections.

I also thank the Bio-Ethics Centre of St. Joseph's College in Edmonton, Alberta for supplying me with reference books and articles on this topic.

A very special thanks to Pastor Max Solbrekken, who helped me in every possible way, to bring this message to the world and to his daughter Betty Farge for coordinating the final manuscript for publishing.

INTRODUCTION

Many articles have been written about the right to die and the legalization of euthanasia. Many surveys have been done amongst health professionals to find out what percentage approve or disapprove of physician-assisted suicide as a means to end someone's suffering. The opinions are divided.[1]

There is also a tendency to make a distinction between *passive euthanasia* and *active euthanasia*. The latter is active in the sense that medication is given to a patient by a doctor, whether or not agreed upon by that patient or his or her family; and the dose is large enough to cause death.

However, more and more cases will be done with the consent of a patient, or his or her family. Living wills will be encouraged by other sources for this purpose. Needless to say, coercion and/or circumstances plays a dominant role here and very little is being done to search for other options in the way of "mercy-killing". It seems technically so simple and straightforward.

Passive euthanasia seems to be a choice for many who recognize that certain diseases have no hope of recovery, or in other cases

---

[1] C.R.S. Dawes, M.D., Letter to the Editor: "Not all Doctors Oppose Euthanasia", *Canadian Medical News*, May 1995, p. 2; and Senate Report: "No legalization for Euthanasia", Canadian Medical Association Journal, July 15, 1995, 153(2), p. 191.

that they will only result in a very poor quality of life. This choice captivates the imagination of both the sufferer and the caregiver. Without further education, it is often, although with great difficulty, a desperate decision towards what appears to be a way of escape, and/or preservation of dignity.

The meaning of passive euthanasia is the withholding of any unnecessary treatment to prolong life in certain patients. *Which patients qualify here?* It usually depends on their age and their condition. Again, living wills (made up by those patients in earlier stages of their disease, containing certain directions as to how far they want treatment to proceed) are very important. Of course, pressure from the family is also important.

What is unnecessary treatment? All kinds of measures are possible here which, if administered to that patient as compared to a younger or healthier one, will result in less desirable effects. It is not hard to conclude then, that rules may vary considerably. More and more exceptions will be presented regarding age and/ or health conditions; whether in positive ways (old but still healthy) or in negative ways (young but wishing to die).

This book is written by a Christian for Christians, and for all who are interested or just curious. *It is not based on philosophy but on Biblical principles.* It will try to dismantle the whole concept of euthanasia, and if possible, even to eliminate it from our options.

I believe euthanasia should be placed back to where it belongs: in Greco-Roman philosophy. As we know, the word "euthanasia" is derived from 'eu' meaning "good" (as in euphoric, a good mood) and 'thanatos' meaning "death". Apparently the Romans did not wait until they were ill or dying; they could at any time choose to die, even during moments of great fame or success, so that they would have only pleasant memories about life. In other words, people could choose to die in an elegant and dignified way, at a time suitable to their taste.

OUR GOD, HOWEVER, IS A GOD OF LIFE, AND IS FULLY CAPABLE OF TAKING US OUT OF THIS LIFE WITHOUT OUR HELP. HE CAN DO IT IN A BEAUTIFUL AND DIGNIFIED WAY!

CHAPTER I

TERMINAL ILLNESS

Terminal illness is a condition which, after being treated with all possible modalities, turns out to be incurable and is slowly or quickly deteriorating towards death. For a better description, it may be easier (when talking about adult patients) to divide terminal illness into the following three stages:

The Initial Stage: The patient has been told the diagnosis and prognosis. Similar to the situation in grief reactions, this stage is characterized by shock, disbelief, denial in the patient and his or her family. Sooner or later, this will be followed by anger, disappointment, and feelings of despair.

The Intermediate Stage: The patient is now undergoing various forms of palliative care, where the main objective is to make him or her comfortable.[2] Emphasis is put on nutrition, fluid balance, pain relief, and bowel and bladder functions. Fresh air and a good environmental temperature is important, along with clean linen sheets, flowers and visits from friends and relatives.

---

[2] N. MacDonald: "Interview re: Aspects of Palliative Care", *Pain Management Newsletter,* Vol. 8, No. 1, April 1995, pp 1-3.

Feelings of despair or depression are waxing and waning, and may intermingle now with the wish to search for other means of healing or relief. There may be efforts made to negotiate with nurses, doctors, or even with God.

The End Stage or Inevitable Stage: The dying process has actually begun. In this stage, the process can be compared to the birth process: certain events will follow one another, one problem will lead to the next. Although medications can definitely slow some processes down, the inevitable next event will come, unless heroic interventions are tried. These will only give "glory" to the one who gives the treatment. The invention of new drugs can sometimes intervene here and give some new hope towards postponement for longer periods of time. But when all of these fail, the dying process continues and can sometimes end in an unexpected way, such as pneumonia, cardiac arrest or multi-organ failure.

In the emotional sphere, there may be acceptance, but there also may still be fear, anger, bitterness and unforgiveness, rebellion, emptiness or even apathy.

R. M. Gula, S.S. writes in his book, *What Are They Saying About Euthanasia?*:

> As the previous chapters show: "Dying" and "terminally ill" are no ironclad categories of some technical sort, and can't be ascertained by clear terms for patients, whose illnesses are progressing towards and likely will cause death within what is to the patient a very short time. Unlike the 'hopelessly ill' patient whose situation is stable and is not progressing towards death, for instance the severely demented or quadriplegic patient, the terminally ill cannot be stabilized, treatment cannot restore the terminally ill to health. Any further medical intervention will only prolong the dying process.

The difficulty of diagnosis and the possibility of surprise recoveries make determining a case of irreversible death or terminal illness difficult. But generally we can make a reasonable estimate that a patient will die in a short time. This reasonable estimate is sufficient for making good moral judgments.[3]

3   R.M. Gula, S.S.: What are They Saying About Euthanasia? (New York: Paulist Press, 1986), p. 137.

CHAPTER II

LIFE AFTER DEATH

A number of books have been written about the "sanctity of life" giving valid reasons why terminally ill patients should be allowed and encouraged to experience a natural death. The questions presented here are: 1) How far should we go, and 2) When will life be a burden, too heavy to carry on?

As we know, the Hippocratic Oath states in A Physician's Pledge: *"I will use treatment to help the sick according to my ability and judgment, but never with a view to injury or wrongdoing. Neither will I administer a poison to anybody when asked to do so, nor will I suggest such a course."* There are clearly shortcomings in this oath pertaining to definitions of injury or wrongdoing. This occurs so often, that those in favour of mercy-killing are convinced they are "helping the sick". They consider death as a desirable form of treatment, and not a poison. They assume that there is no need for spiritual preparedness before death to ensure their "blessed eternal state". To them, death ends everything.

IS THERE REALLY NOTHING AFTER DEATH, or does life continue in a different way? Is there a soul or spirit, and should we not rather discuss 'the sanctity of the soul' rather than the questionable 'sanctity of life'? Again, numerous philosophies and religions have their own speculations about life after death. There is no definite proof that "nothing will follow after death"!

How do we cope with the uncertainty regarding existence after death? And how do we change during the days of terminal illness?

Reverend George Tattrie writes in his book *Euthanasia: A Christian Perspective*, that the Greek saw mercy-killing as acceptable and prevalent in their culture because illness was considered a curse and a healthy mind can only exist in a healthy body.[4] Several coping mechanisms are derived from Greek culture or other religions; or they can originate from the individual's lifestyle:

A) Denial of negative outcomes after death. This concept generalizes that regardless of each individual's lifestyle or behaviour, death will be a deliverance from curses and illnesses. Denial also denies the triune composition of the human being and that spirit and soul are separated from the body at death. There is also a denial of any form of judgment, since the Greeks were polytheists and believed in many gods instead of One True God. They dealt with spiritual matters through mythology.

B) Rationalization is another coping mechanism. Its purpose is to help the individual adjust and comprehend the outcome after death. One example is the Buddhist teaching that *nihilism* follows death, or *reincarnation*, or the *transition* into another second human life with similar features like the present one. These and other religions' coping mechanisms will ultimately mean a separation of the dying person from his or her loved ones. The dying person will either go to an unknown place,

---

[4]   Rev. G. Tattrie: Euthanasia, A Christian Perspective, (Don Mills, Ontario: Board of Congregational Life, The Presbyterian Church in Canada, 1982), p. 1.

or disappear into nothingness where no future reunion with loved ones is possible.

Death for these individuals then, is a necessary evil, and should be made as comfortable as possible to ease the pain for all persons involved. They see dying as an unnecessarily painful process which has no meaning and should be shortened if possible.

Dying means destruction and can occur in ugly ways, or artificially "improved" ways when so desired.

C) Repression of feelings, relying on pride. One has to pretend that man can control his own destiny, so death should be faced without fear or complaints. This attitude may create feelings of loneliness and "longing for the end".

D) Substitution: Trying to diminish fears and decrease doubts by obtaining material objects for comfort.

E) Open rebellion: Anger is used to fight the controversy of death. Of course, any of these can occur in combinations together.

For a Christian, it is possible to stand on a firm foundation based on promises by God as the only Higher Power, Who knows how to love His creation, and especially to love human beings who were created in His image.

WILL HE, WHO IS ETERNAL, NOT CREATE US AS ETERNAL SOULS? AND IF WE ARE ETERNAL, WILL THERE NOT BE AN ETERNAL RESIDENCE WHERE WE WILL ALL BE REUNITED?

Christians do believe in positive or negative outcomes and a first judgment, where souls will be rewarded in heaven, or stay in Sheol (Hades). Later there will be a final judgment, and an exodus of lost souls towards the lake of fire, or second death.

But Christians also believe that God has given us a free will to choose between those two destinations, and to act on it according to principles outlined in the Bible!

CHAPTER III

PAIN AND SUFFERING, ARE THEY LIMITLESS?

With these issues in mind, we wonder whether it is true that certain pains are "uncontrollable" during certain illnesses? Is suffering through feelings of deep depression or worthlessness really unavoidable? Are there really deaths without dignity, and is there nothing that can be done? Is there one factor, or is there a combination of any or all of these factors, that create such a fear in the terminally ill person, that that person feels compelled to think about other ways to avoid those dreadful events?

If the outcome is death any way, can death be altered to make it more acceptable? Is it easier for those standing at the bedside to watch someone going into a deep sleep followed by death, or to watch someone in agony, gasping, or comatose? These and more dilemmas undoubtedly fill the minds of those favouring euthanasia.

Let us read a letter of a man who, even when he was not sure of what to expect, already made his point clear: He did not want "a cup of poison."

I am a layman. Some time ago I read your guest editorial by Dr. Stephen and Shelagh Genuis, titled "Living and Dying with Dignity" in the June edition of your Journal (of Obstetrics and Gynaecology). I took particular interest in this article because I am disabled with the chronic degenerative disease multiple sclerosis (MS). It seems that the world is getting so bleak for people like me, with talk of euthanasia and "death and dignity". The Genuis' editorial allowed me to imagine the world as more inviting. It was a welcome contrast to the starkness of the "death and dignity" philosophy which seemed so . . . well, . . . stark. Thank you, Dr. Stephen and Shelagh Genuis. Our world needs more people like you.

When I developed MS and my own health began slipping away for want of an effective treatment, I wondered about a world that would offer me death with dignity at my lowest point and overwhelmed with grief. I did not need somebody standing beside me to offer death with dignity. No! I needed somebody standing beside me committed to finding a life with dignity even if I ceased to desire it. It was not the time for granting death-wishes. Is it ever?

My mind is filled with so many questions! Is it mere coincidence of timing that Canada is talking of a mounting health care crisis while discussions on euthanasia and doctor assisted suicide are on the rise? And with all this discussion of doctor assisted suicide, I also wonder what doctors think? After all, they are the ones who will be asked to shift their role from healers to executioners. Does the medical profession want this? (Apparently the medical profession does not want this, according to a recent CMA vote.) And what of us potential recipients—the chronically or terminally ill? Will the right to die with dignity eventually become the duty to die with dignity? What will my society evolve into if it accepts euthanasia, death with dignity, and the noting that some lives are not worthy to be lived? Will I want to live in such a society—a society that has ceased to see itself as nurturing?

Acceptance of euthanasia for us (the chronically or terminally ill) is our ultimate isolation, our ultimate exclusion, our ultimate rejection. The heavy-hearted, the suicidal, and the vulnerable need the human family's embrace—its love—its acceptance—not a poisoned cup cleverly disguised under a veil of compassion. Forget the poverty of the personal autonomy myth! We are community. We are interdependent, not dependent. This is the underlying truth that I believe the Genuis' editorial addressed. The goal must never be the hopelessness of so-called "death and dignity", rather the affirmation of searching for life and dignity. Our nation needs more people with the wisdom of Dr. Stephen and Shelagh Genuis. Thank you.

Yours sincerely,
Mark Pickup, Beaumont, Alberta[5]

Dr. Harvey M. Chochinov writes about "The Five D's" of fears in cancer patients:

Death: concerns about one's own vulnerability, mortality, and the fate of those one would leave behind.

Disability: fear of being unable to carry out prior designated roles, e.g. worker, provider, lover, partner, parent, etc.

Disfigurement: a worry especially in those with head and neck malignancies, breast cancer, genito-urinary cancers and those requiring ostomies.

---

[5] M. Pickup: "Letters to the editor", *Journal Society of Obstetrics and Gynaecology Canada*, March 1995, pp. 229-230.

Dependence: loss of control and having to depend on others for care, which is a common concern and cause of much distress among cancer patients.

Loss of Desirability: patients fear losing everyone they hold most dear: While this has implication in terms of sexual life, it also may take the form of fearing abandonment by family, friends and even health care providers.[6]

"These are certainly serious aspects of emotional suffering and the patient may need help from a psycho-oncologist. While the above five D's are indeed normal, they can be profoundly distressing, painful and disruptive. In fact, emotional suffering is among the least studied and most poorly understood components of the subjective cancer experience. With understanding, patience and empathy from health care providers, those responses usually resolve within two to three weeks as the patient adjusts to new information, confronts the issues presented, finds reasons for optimism, and resumes activities such as new or revised treatment plans."[7]

As incredible as it seems, in palliative care it is possible to control cancer pain to a tolerable degree by the use of continuous subcutaneous infusion of analgesics, or else with nebulized morphine8/. or with fentanyl patches.

An interesting article by J.M. Jones, R.N. describes a video about effective pain management in small, rural communities, when health care professionals team up to facilitate palliative pain strategies and care. Community palliative care and home care

---

6   H. M. Chochinov, M.D., F.R.C.P.C.: "Psychiatric Care of the Cancer Patient", *Medicine*, North America, Nov/Dec 1994, pp. 671-674.

7   H. M. Chochinov, M.D. F.R.C.P.C.: "Treating Depression in the Terminally Ill, *Pain Management Newsletter, supra*, note 1, pp. 4-5.

work together to give the patient a painfree "at home" life.9/. The article says further: "During the initial stages of terminal illness, the patient can return to many of his/her usual activities at home as that person regains a "reason to live" 10/.

Are there deaths without dignity? When we consider the five D's as mentioned by Chochinov, there are factors contributing to the lack of dignity, and they should be corrected although not by induction of death. When the factors of severe pain, emotional suffering and uncertainty regarding the illness or life after death are all present, the dying person often perceives death as the only solution. Do we, as caregivers, share their uncertainty?

The following is an interesting description by a medical student entitled: "DYING.: A POSITIVE RATHER THAN A NEGATIVE EXPERIENCE".

"One of the things I had always thought was that patients who were facing a terminal illness wouldn't want to live." McCorquodale says to her surprise, she soon learned that the opposite was in fact the case. Although the patients go through their anger, grief, and denial, they reach a point where they are accepting of [their situations] and are glad to just be alive. If you can control somebody's pain and discomfort as well as their nausea and other symptoms they can find a reason to live.

McCorquodale had imagined that a palliative care service might be a depressing place; in fact the prevailing atmosphere was one of hope. *"It was very positive—very uplifting"* she notes, adding that *"there was more time to share with friends and family. I was particularly impressed by both the teamwork and the amount of time spent with patients letting them work through what it feels like to be dying, instead of just "how did you sleep?" or "how have you been eating?"*

At the same time, *McCorquodale* saw that this close level of contact with patients could also exact an emotional toll from caregivers. There was one case which she can recall well; it was that of a teenage girl with a devastating brain malignancy. She was very ill, having a lot of pain and other symptoms. Dealing with her was such a struggle, *McCorquodale* remembers with an intense sadness. *"We all had a lot of trouble. It was difficult not to identify with her—somebody young who was dying rather than an older patient. It seemed less normal. Various members of the team were having a really hard time, yet we were able to support each other through it. When she died, it was sad but we were all relieved for her."*

HOW CAN WE BEST SUSTAIN HOPE? Speaking to the question of how best to sustain hope, *McCorquodale* points to the critical role of the emotional component of suffering. *"I think that it is immense. Those patients I saw who were without hope, who experienced the most pain and suffering were those who were alone. They either had language or cultural barriers, and so were unable to communicate with us."* In a significant observation revealing much about the fundamental nature of both hope and suffering, the single two instances where she encountered patients who had lost the will to live were those without any family and *"attributed their wish to die to isolation."*

While *McCorquodale* acknowledges that the palliative care philosophy may at first blush seem to run contrary to traditional medical precepts, she believes that the truth lies somewhere beyond this perspective. *"For the most part, we are all afraid of dying. We've been trained to guard against death—to do everything we can in preventing it. Having seen these patients die, I don't feel as much fear [of death] when it has come naturally. Even where pain is controlled, in the end, dying becomes a positive rather then a negative experience."*[11]

WHAT ARE LIVING WILLS, AND WILL THEY BE HELPFUL? Dr. Peter Singer, a Toronto internist, Associate Professor of Medicine and Associate Director of the University of Toronto Centre for Bioethics stated:

Sometimes called advance directives, a living will guides future health care when you may be too ill to make decisions about the kind of care you want. It is filled out when you are competent or capable and takes effect when you are incapable of expressing your wishes, It is separate from a standard will which directs the distribution of property after death.[12]

Dr. Singer further states: "Through advance care planning and knowing people's preferences, death can be more peaceful.[13] I think that living wills will be very helpful to maintain dignity during the dying process [although the patient may need some help from counsellors or loved ones].

A living will includes:

A list of common conditions [e.g. mild, moderate, or severe stroke or dementia, permanent coma, terminal illness] and a list of common treatments [e.g. CPR, ventilator, dialysis, life-saving surgery, tube-feeding]. "Yes, no, undecided, or treatment trial" should be checked off for each combination of health situation and treatment. Other instructions express personal care decisions about shelter, nutrition, clothing, and hygiene.[14] Pg. 14 [in the original document]

Being a caregiver, one has to be aware of all these circumstances, and understand that in many cases, the ill person has not been told, or does not believe that help is possible in a real way. Some of them may become confused because of the sedative effect of certain medications and may have to be positively encouraged in their spirits while the mind is clouded.

As a caregiver one has to diligently continue to search for other methods to provide that help. A few years ago, the concept of hospice care gained popularity. THE PRINCIPLES FOR HOSPICE CARE INCLUDE HELPING AND CARING WHERE CURING IS NOT POSSIBLE ANYMORE. Hospice care is palliative care of the highest quality with maximum control of pain and suffering, to prepare spirit, soul and body for the transition into eternity.

During hospice care one should not say "Go in peace" which may indicate "I don't really care, you may decide for yourself".

Instead, we must ask: "How can we make you more comfortable, what else can we do to show you our undying love?" Here I would like to quote from an article by Dr. B. Mount: "Eradicate the suffering, not the sufferer."[15]

Dr. Mount also writes about a patient who requested euthanasia. The question was: "Would competent palliative care have controlled Mrs. Solomon's physical suffering? Almost certainly. Would palliative care have been successful in assisting her to achieve her need to be in control? Probably, particularly if the palliative care team, having attended to physical, psycho-social and spiritual needs, and having ruled out depression, acknowledged the importance of mental anguish and decided with patient and family that sedation to the point of comfort will always be a viable option. Or, one can regard the palliative care as a catalyst to a new-found ability to accommodate to increasing dependency.[16]

CHAPTER IV

WHAT IS AGGRESSIVE COMPASSIONATE CARE?

Compassion originates from >com= meaning "together", and >passion= meaning "suffering", so in the combined form we understand what the meaning is: *"suffering together"*. The caregiver should place himself or herself in the same situation as the ill person, and try to understand the ill person, and then try to support that person as much as possible.

Are feelings of pity unavoidable? And are such feelings appropriate or should one try to hide them? Can we do more than just feel this way and only try to make them feel physically comfortable? Is there a possibility of reversing the negative experiences and turn them into positive ones, as previously described by the medical student in the Pain Management Newsletter?[17] Is it possible to determine the stage of the illness in order to act accordingly?

I think that it is important to study hospice care.[18] The mission of a hospice is to care for the terminally ill and their families: the focus for hospice is on life and the alleviation of suffering.[19] The goal of euthanasia, on the other hand, is to create "a good death" by administering a quick-acting drug or by withholding vital necessities in order to promote death. I do not believe that a good death can only be achieved by euthanasia. Although in hospice care, life is the focus, a good and peaceful death must certainly be kept in mind., and one must work towards this goal.

Dr. I.R. Byock speaks about "a more assertive approach", and insists that "physical suffering among the dying is unnecessary". *"Hospice philosophy is not only compatible with an energetic, assertive approach to terminal symptom management, it demands it".*[20]

This is not always easy, and may not be complete either. Intensive intervention is necessary at the final stages, but also during day-to-day care, based upon our understanding of the state of the soul of each person we are dealing with.

Senator Keon, a Roman Catholic, is concerned about the clandestine use of euthanasia in recent years. He states that five percent of terminally ill patients do not want palliative care as they understand it, or as they have witnessed it in people they know of, mostly for fear of loss of autonomy.[21] Questions that naturally arise are: Is there fear because of lack of information, or is the patient actually in open rebellion?

He agrees that it is important to be pro-active in the end-of-life management and try to care for the terminally ill in such a way as to "ease the dying process" and to prevent unnecessary prolongation of death.[22]

Dr. N. Nazerali writes about "a rapidly evolving trend to encourage seniors to express advance health care directives". I would suggest here to *use sound Biblical principles* and that the "physicians will be required to master the art of guiding patients to making autonomous decisions". In certain patients where no close family is present to take care of them, additional team work is necessary to provide the important care and counselling.

It is my personal opinion that there is what we may call "the dying process", which is a final stage of the last in terminal illness. I see this as a turning point manifested as irreversible, progressive deterioration. In a certain sense it is *comparable to the birthing process,* where clearly there are true contractions of the womb instead of "false labour". In the dying process there is a true and clear loss of function in vital organs, leading to cessation of life. It is in this stage that acceptance of death can take place; and it is in this stage that any intervention with the aim of restoring to a previous stage is disruptive, such as would be understandable in the birthing process. These unnatural interventions are often termed "futile" or "totally ineffective" instead of "disruptive". *My opinion is that a peaceful death without further intervention is the natural course to be followed,* and this natural process is preferable as compared to calculations and discussions regarding usefulness or effectiveness or "quality of life". The giving of comfort should generally be accepted as the standard for determining the level of care in final stages. This standard of "comfort" is compatible with the quotation from Senator Keon answers, i.e. *"To comfort is to ease the dying process".*

To ease the dying process, then, means trying to make the transition from one stage to the next as smoothly as possible; and to aim at the highest quality of comfort for the dying person involved. If at all possible, the caregivers should induce feelings of joy and peace. From these care-givers should come an attitude of overcoming or encouragement, as a basis for counselling and caring.

The Bible describes *"overcoming"* in many texts [referring to eagles, conquerors, kings, priests, and ambassadors] and by using these texts one is enabled to offer a level of care which is more than basic palliative care; this is what I call *"aggressive compassionate care".* One can see this as positively directed, confrontational, compassionate care for the whole person, not just a dying body and a withering soul.

One has to be alert at all times and be aware of the journey of the soul with regards to its destination. One can be reassured that there is no reason to interrupt anything; either forwards [promoting quicker death] or backwards [postponing death] because by slowly and humbly following natural events, one is working actively to achieve not only a good death, but possibly the highest quality of death, i.e. a peaceful transition into eternal life!

There is no doubt that family or loved ones can be included in the above type of care,[24] because this will help them in the grieving process after departure. There will then be agreement about reunion and togetherness forever.

A very interesting article was written by Dr. John F. Scott, Director of the Regional Palliative Care Services in Ottawa and Head of Palliative Medicine at the University of Ottawa, after he presented his brief to the Parliamentary Committee. He spoke against Bill C-203, and he clearly outlined the meaning of palliative care. He said that *Canadians must not believe the lie* that they are faced with a choice between a quick, good death and a slow painful one.[26]

He emphasized that additional legal protection is required to decrease inappropriate "over-treatment" and to encourage palliative care. He acknowledged that at the root of pain, palliative care is fear, misunderstanding and a sense of helplessness. He certainly encourages discussion at length with patient, family and health care team.[27]

He mentions further that consent for therapy withdrawal can be neither free nor informed unless one of the alternatives offered is *active palliative care*, in which not only are symptoms relieved, but there are resources and time available for compassionate personalized care.[28]

CHAPTER V

WHY EUTHANASIA IS NOT AN OPTION IN PALLIATIVE CARE.

After all of the reflections in the previous chapters, we may conclude that "euthanasia" is actually a misnomer if one wants to indicate *"mercy-killing"* or *"letting die because of despair"*. Both of the latter phrases indicate acts of violence, [one is overt, the other is covert] whereas "euthanasia" only means "a good death" in its literal sense. Death may appear as something desirable, something dignified, to be preferred above an insurmountable, indescribable suffering with no end in sight, and a suffering that seems to be senseless . . .

But why does it have to be to be by violence, disguised by soft words, as if compassion is the motive? In fact, it is more likely that uncertainty, insecurity, anxiety, self-remorse, and being overwhelmed, are the real motives. These feelings are not only very possible in a patient, but also in the caregiver, since "compassion" means that they are "suffering together". I strongly suggest that in the role of a caregiver one should try to be more pro-active, and certainly be more aware of one's own anxieties, and work to overcome them. Be aware also of all the circumstances and reasons for the prolongation and complexity of the process in certain people.

Most of us who believe in the *existence of a spirit and soul within human beings*, will agree that a holistic approach, based on attention to body, soul and spirit is necessary during the preservation of life, as well as during the preparation for transition into eternal life. We will agree that death only means a cessation of physical life, but by no means is it a total termination of spiritual life. Is it not surprising that there seems to be a parallel between the questions around the beginning of life and those around the so called end of life. There is a tendency towards looking for the obvious signs rather than searching for the actual truth.

In the care of an aging population and certain groups of seriously ill patients it is often seen that that there is a slower decline over a longer period with a lengthy period of disability and, of course, more complex physical and psycho-spiritual problems.[29] Also because of increased mobility in society, families may live too far away, neighbours may not know each other; therefore a dying person can be quite lonely and lacking practical and emotional support. Thus, there is a need for a more noble and credible place for suffering people; there is also a need for more support and respite for caregivers to prevent them from ending up in various "burn-out" and stress-syndromes.

Euthanasia, if translated into "good death" should be a peaceful transition from earthly life according to natural rules without any type of violence, induction or self-infliction; *a peaceful death that will acknowledge God's authority and sovereignty over natural laws.* The transition should take place in dignified surroundings, with full expectancy of a glorious arrival in the "Promised Land", which is described in the Bible as having "streets of gold" and "gates of pearl". When this full acceptance is a reality in the dying person, no form of violent assistance is needed. If not naturally present, any imposed interruption is dangerous for the soul in journey.

IN OTHER WORDS, DEATH-INDUCING INTERVENTIONS ARE UNNECESSARY AND SHOULD BE ABOLISHED FOREVER!

In conclusion then, we can say that the dying process, although perceived as a crisis, can become a journey of joy instead of a frightening experience. In this journey, travelers go through the process together, while the dying person can see a clear goal in front of him/her. Shortcuts are not possible on this *"straight and narrow way"* to eternity. Worse still, those shortcuts may change the transition from a bright one into a dark one or into another eternity, which represents a total separation from God.

What if the dying individual is unconscious, or in the case of an infant, unable to communicate or to share feelings? What if there is cognitive failure?[30] Soul and mind can be disconnected in this way, but the spirit is more alive, and is capable of agreeing with our prayers, whether or not we ask for further progression, or for combat in spiritual warfare against hindering spirits. [this topic will be discussed again in chapter V when we look at the prolonged dying process and at those who are in the vegetative state]

DEATH, if celebrated as a successful achievement through obedience and submission to natural laws, is a totally different concept from the original proposal in Greco-Roman philosophy, where man had power over life and death. In fact, we read in the Bible that the power to give and take life does not belong to man, no matter what motives there may be. This is not a question of "sanctity of life" but of the sovereignty of God. Of paramount importance is the understanding of the existence of spirit, soul and body.[31] A successful and peaceful death can become a valuable help for surviving relatives, who have to go through the bereavement process.

I wrote this small booklet because of the many openly *publicized acts of euthanasia on television and in articles.* It is my conviction that every effort should be made to replace euthanasia with a structured compassionate care based on acknowledgement and full respect for the spirit, soul and body as one unified entity!

CHAPTER VI

RETURN TO DUST OR TO GLORY?

[This is a personal meditation about our eternal spirits, followed by some useful reports and suggestions for palliative care].

When Heaven comes to earth, referring to Jesus' prayer to His Father: *"Your Will be done in earth as it is in Heaven"*, and both become one, death will no longer be necessary! I believe that this will happen, and that at such a time, God's Will will be done, just like Jesus' words in the first 'Our Father', which is now known as 'the Lord's Prayer'.

For Heaven and earth, this represents the perfect union, similar to the situation in Eden; in other words it will be a return of the same Paradise where Adam and Eve lived.

This happens initially, when we are born again by the Word of God and the Holy Spirit. His will then begins to be done in this earth—our bodies!

Prior to our birth as human beings, and before the foundations of the world, we were already known by God and predestined to be His children. (Eph. 1:3-6) And since our spirits came from God (Eccl. 12:7), we may have been aware of a real heaven and it stands to reason that we would continue to long for that place!

Through the New Birth, however, we receive regenerated spirits and are filled with the Almighty Holy Spirit of God! (Titus 3:5; Acts 2:4)

The Bible says that even now, *"we are seated together in heavenly places in Christ"*. (Eph. 2:6)

The psalmist in Ps. 103 wrote: "Bless the Lord, oh my soul, and forget not all His benefits, Bless His Holy Name! How I would like to add now: "Bless the Lord's creation [the earth], bless all the beauty of His creation, bless all that can make us cry for joy, and long for more!"

When death comes near, I wonder if the dying person can see some of this Heaven to earth phenomenon. As we all know, Heaven is where God the Father is, with Jesus at His right hand. The dying person is about to be changed or "translated", and may see no difference between one step and the other into eternity.

I will give some examples to clarify what I mean by certain statements about Heaven's perfection and man's possible, episodic awareness of this perfection.

First example: the knowledge of beauty can only be possible if we ever have possessed the concept or the understanding of: the ultimate beauty, the beauty beyond comparison, the beauty beyond description, the perfect beauty, without spots or wrinkles. Only then can we look at God's creation, and say that one thing is as beautiful, or more beautiful than something else.

Second example: the feeling of joy and perfection, and the looking forward to it, can only be understood if we have felt and sensed during life on earth, mountaintops, the ends of the earth, the inner fire by the Holy Spirit [when we are filled with the Holy Spirit], extremely joyful, or overflowing [abundant, more than usual] sensations. In this scenario, our impressions are pointing to a glorious future, in eternity. Shall we then compare this with what the Bible describes as "joys unspeakable"? Can we say that we would like to try this or that activity in order to generate joy that might come close to the perfect joy in Heaven, when realizing our glorious nature.

Third example: the longing to possess something, is only comprehensible after we were in possession of the total fullness of the soul and spirit, the abundance as a standard measurement, the total satisfaction and fulfilment, [so that every other request will become painful and undesirable], and finally: the eternal riches in glory (Phil. 4: 19).

Fourth example: the longing to achieve, to conquer, to surpass, is comprehensible only if once we were: without boundaries, soaring like eagles, possessing youth which is renewable, and being totally fearless. *[Our spirits were once perfect, and now we are temporarily restricted]*.

Fifth example: feelings for harmony and wellness can only be explained if we ever have existed in the fullness of *Zoe*, the source of life where all fractions work together for one purpose: fulfilling the will of God. If we understood that the "balm of Gilead" as described in the Bible, was something real for us, and that healing and harmony were indistinguishable concepts. Because of these, the *Oil of Joy* was flowing abundantly, and the garments of Praise were used daily, to praise Him for His Mercy. It is understood that the garments of praise were to be used to celebrate the victory already won by Jesus, and that He is the "I am" [past, present, future] and what was won will still represent victory, and will show more victory in the future. *The garments of praise* can be a sign of the task of an ambassador in Christ [2 Cor, 5:20]; they represent "Excellence for Jesus", and just before the Rapture we will be recognized as His children because of the garments we wear at that time.

To make it clear: we will show our colours, proclaim our beliefs, and our faith-foundation according to Heb. 11:1. We do not have to see to believe, but we believe and stand on His promises, and we will then see the manifestations!

To re-iterate once more I repeat: we were, at one time, real spirits, now living in a body. We will remain spirits, when leaving the body. Thus, the return to dust is applicable to our bodies only, and our spirits will move into a new dimension, which in the Bible is called "glorified bodies". (Romans 8:29-30)

Having said all this, in what way can a dying person focus on these thoughts and be able to feel joy and interest? Feel dignified? Having no thoughts of disintegration?

A) Most important issue for all care-givers is the knowledge and the full usage of all methods of pain-management, [E.J.Latimer, 1996][29]. We must consider easing the pains and controlling all symptoms leading to pain and discomfort, such as confusion and difficulties with breathing. Also important are the feelings of depression and loneliness in certain patients, and the awareness of disfigurement or mutilation in others. Restlessness or delirium can be treated, mouth-ulcers and yeast-infections should be attended to as good as possible.

A difficult issue comes up when we have to face "emotional pains" [Yves Quenneville, 1996][39] Here we may feel inside ourselves the tendency to withdraw, or to maintain stubborn optimism, or to speak hollow phrases. We have to understand that the patient needs some sense of control.

We should not forget to consider "total pain" [S. Lawrence Librach, 1995][19], which includes personality, family issues, and neuropathic pains.

B) There are many controversial matters in palliative care [Paul S. Links, 1998][37]. A suicidal person is actually ambivalent; a passion for life often co-exists with despair. Some are using thoughts of death to cope with life. Hope and despair and renewal often exist side by side.

My comment on this is, that the care-giver should be strong during these expressions of despair, knowing that feelings of hope will return. Another problem is to determine when to withhold or withdraw treatment or nutrition. Most experts will say: *"Only when continuation of either one causes physiologically harmful changes"*.

C) The terminally ill often needs counselling and regular communication. Questions often asked are: "How can I control my situation, and why can I not choose my own preferred way of dying?" [K.G. Wilson & ass. April 1998][40].

In Dutch surveys it has been found that most of their patients really fear their "loss of dignity" or "unworthy dying", "being dependent on others" and even just being "tired of life".

PAIN is seldom the predominant reason . . . Depression, if present, is known to be potentially treatable [K.G. Wilson] and [H.M. Chochinov] 1996[31]. One should see treatment more as a way to lift depression, because depression in itself is a psycho-spiritual condition, and counselling should go hand-in-hand with the correction of neuro-transmitters.

Are personal directives necessary? What about the competency of the ill person? [R. Heydemann, 1997][33]. Or in cases of delirium, should the individual be declared ineligible to complete a personal directive? It stands to reason, that without a personal directive made in advance, the family will feel dis-empowered. The physician in charge has to balance his decisions between the law and compassion. Says one family physician, M. Addison.[1] "The benefit of personal directives is that they formalize communication".

D) Yes, nutrition is very important, in questions like: "How much, and how long"?

Nutrition is considered as minimal care and will have to be readjusted often according to the strength of the body and the stage of the dying process. [W.A. Lafrance, 1997][34]. It really is not comparable to medical treatments, because some of the latter can become disproportional. Nevertheless, in certain terminal cases, nutrition can be harmful too, and should be replaced with fluids only to prevent dehydration.

E) Care and respect are needed under all circumstances. The issue of *"preserving someone's dignity"* should have top priority.

CHAPTER VII

SHADOW OF THE METAPHORS

In this chapter we will look at, what seems like "the inability to die" or in more logical terms: "the prolonged dying process". This event may happen, when the dying process has started, but does not progress as expected, and even may look like the process has arrested. In a survey regarding opinions from a community in Singapore, most of them feared to have to go through this.[38]

A clear example [to my understanding], is the recent case of Dr. N. Morrison from Halifax; she tried to relieve pain in a patient, [Paul Wills]. He remained alive, after his life support was removed. While he was clearly in a dying process, death would not take place, at least not according to the usual observations and standards.[44]

Many questions may arise here: "When is a long course too long?" "What is the cause of this?" "Should it always be treated, and by what method?" "How much pain is in a patient who is unconscious?" "What is agony?" "Since when is a lethal dose of a non-analgesic drug appropriate for someone in a dying process?"

I can imagine that the impression of the judge was: "There was no intention to kill". But there could perhaps be other reasons for the action, such as personal ambivalence, feelings of horror and dismay, feelings of despair and powerlessness, or in other cases: the reluctance to consult spiritual informants or experts. The same feelings were obviously in the nurse also, who spoke about the patient as an "indestructible" man.

In fact, there were certain cases known in The Netherlands, who failed to die despite the usual lethal doses of narcotics; and many needed to be paralysed in their respiratory muscles, to secure death, [this was shown in a TV-program}.

The article about the Halifax case goes further, saying that animals are being treated better, indicating that the writer has no concepts about soul, spirit and body, or eternal life; in other words, she considers them as metaphors. Therefore, there is indeed no hope for someone who considers the Bible full of metaphors.

Metaphors are [according to the Webster Dictionary] *transfer issues, to be carried; a figure of speech which is founded on resemblance, a word is transferred from an object to which properly belongs, to another in such a manner that a comparison is implied though not formerly expressed.*

A body which is unable to die, may contain a soul in bondage, shadowed by metaphors which ruled during its life. Whether there are spiritual or physical bonds, is unknown, and these are not described in regular journals. If the person is a non-believer, chances are that scriptures in the Bible were seen as metaphors.

A PERSON WHO BELIEVES IN METAPHORS AND COMPLETELY DISREGARD ANY TRUTHS FROM THE BIBLE FACES A SENSELESS DEATH! The stages of grief, as established by E. Kubler-Ross, will be maximised and mixed with feelings of wondering and questioning, rationalizing and trials towards cold reasoning. Indeed there will be no hope for the dying person, if there is no understanding about resurrection *[Re-incarnation seems like a poor surrogate].* I really think that metaphors are among the hindrances blocking the focus during the dying process. There are not too many explanations in recent medical journals about these "prolonged dying cases". Some were written by authors regarding prolonged vegetative states or comas.

COHEN wrote about creating a good quality of death, [prompt, predictable and comfortable] which was achieved by[35] discontinuation of kidney-dialysis in patients considered to be deteriorating too much. "Quality of death" was rated on scales of 1-5 according to duration of dying, discomfort and psycho-social circumstances. I would suggest the question here: Is end-stage renal disease considered a dying process at a certain stage, for instance when other organs fail? Or should the person be discontinued long before that point, so that he/she can still spend some valuable time with the relatives? It certainly is a bio-ethical dilemma. I still think that more studies are necessary.

FREEMAN wrote about "exits from prolonged persistent coma/ vegetative states".[37] Many of these posttraumatic states are unpredictable and can easily fall into decisions to withdraw treatment or to stop nutrition. An article by ANDREAS, K. et al from Austria, reported the use of an MRI-scan to predict with fair accuracy the outcome of those states. [PVS means posttraumatic vegetative states].

In conclusion: An inability to die is a prolonged dying process with no logical explanation, and thus remains a difficult dilemma for caregivers. Organic causes are difficult to determine, there are no studies available. Spiritually there are many questions to be answered. Scriptures which may be important are the ones regarding the resurrection of Lazarus.

Jesus stated that "Lazarus's illness is not unto death, but for the glory of God" [despite the fact that he had been in the grave for 4 days]; In other words, Lazarus was not on his way home yet. [John 11:4]

Perhaps it is more important to look at the physical/organic responses of the body while giving nutrition or medications, and the body will indicate the stage of the dying process. For example, intravenous nutrition may not be effective anymore because of poor circulation.

Jewish medical ethics are strongly pro-life [COHEN],[32] However, also here are limits.

When ethical conflicts arise, the physician may choose to consult a knowledgeable rabbi for a ruling. If the ruling conflicts with the civil law, the latter always prevail and the doctor must refer the patient to another competent physician who does not feel bound by rabbinic authority.

Advance directives are again very important in prolonged dying.[43] They should be discussed and explained long before the time of dying; perhaps as part of making a testament or last will.

One must explain the meaning of choices between withholding or withdrawing treatment or nutrition. These advance directives should be accessible and accompanied by a person as a backup or appropriate proxy.

A few years have passed since chapter seven and addendum. My disease has progressed to using a wheelchair regularly and twenty-four-hour care in a residual. Therefore I decided to update the book, especially because euthanasia is still illegal for everyone. Unfortunately, there are many cases of people with or without depression who are given pills by their doctor to keep at home, with the understanding that they may take the pills if they want to end their lives

CHAPTER VIII

HOW TO FIGHT THE ENEMY

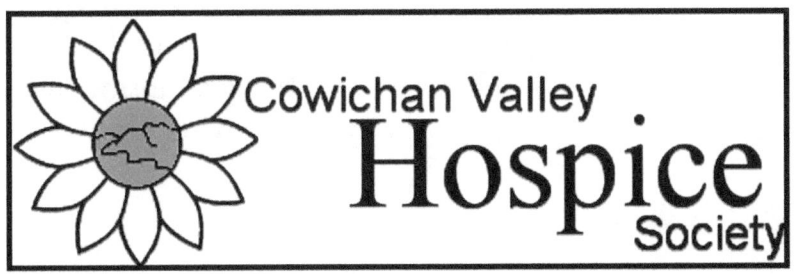

In 1950 understanding for hospices became more acceptable, meaning that "the dying need a different approach". In the mid-60's Dr. Elizabeth Kubler-Ross wrote in her book "Death and dying", a clear explanation about grief, and what is involved when it happens during death and dying and terminal illness. The new concept at that time was hospices, which are places for palliative care, that with a general background of silence. In fact in the hospice the patient has special and different care after the normal treatments have been stopped. The goal is optimal comfort and relief from any pressure or discomfort. Changes in goal and destination may differ for each person, but for all, dignity must be maintained. Human fears should be minimized and all pains should be decreased as much as possible by decreasing memories of pain. In other words, pain medications by injection before the next pain starts. Heart and lungs will be given general supported care, digestive system will get regular fluids to maintain daily balance eventually may be given hypodermoclysis. Communication must be maintained using daily reports between the workers and psychologist and/or social worker.

Why Aggressive? There should be a difference between aggressiveness and only hoping, because one must keep in mind that no measures are impossible and everything should be used in optimal way; no restrictions. In conclusion, there is a heavy emphasis on prayer, and what to expect the prayer should be showing respect towards the person's religion, might be person to person or together with family. There should be clear, specific requests, not only general words, the requests can be large or small, significant or insignificant, for instance decrease of pain, better breathing. Again the difference of aggressive or normal that there is a clear goal inside, relentless attitudes in prayer, based on faith/ or other divine promises . . .

Reference: Cowichan Valley Hospice Society

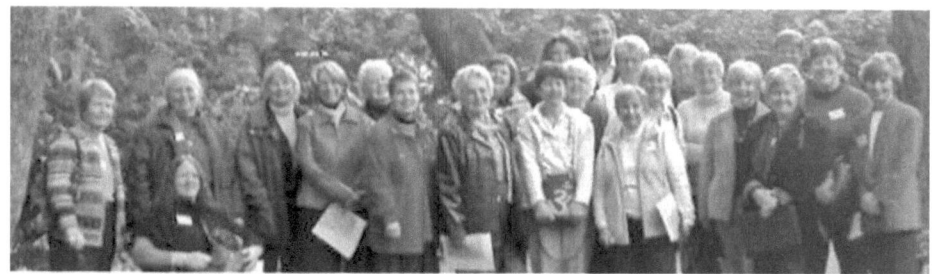

Volunteers

Based on John 15:16

Lover of my soul, I thank you for choosing me here on earth. Thank you for taking me from where I was standing in a crowd. You embraced me and told me that You wanted to write my name in the Book of Life, not because of anything I did, but by Your grace alone and my surrender to You.

By choosing me, You have beautified the deepest parts of my soul, such as I never have experienced before. I feel highly valued, highly preferred, highly desired, and intensely loved, totally one in the spirit with You.

Thank You Jesus, for giving me this vision in a dream!

August, 1995

Addendum for 2006, regarding the sad case of TERRY SCHIAFO, her husband and parents. Terminal events, 15 years before, were anorexia, electrolyte imbalance, cardiac arrest despite resuscitation. Her brain remained in a vegetative state for the next 15 yrs

Parents were under the impression that some speech therapy and rehab were attempted and remained strongly opposed against the removal of her feeding tube; finally the case was decided in favor of a late natural death i.e. removal of the tubefeedings.

We learn that in all uncertain cases a total honesty is needed, from parents, siblings, spouses, and the medical profession

CHAPTER IX

THE MOST DIFFICULT CASES
(see addendum at the end of book 1)

BE STRONG (2)

Persistent vegetative state or syndrome:

This is one of the most difficult cases to be faced by a hospice worker. This is because there are many causes for the disease. Most of them are caused by trauma or toxic substances; occur in all ages and appear to the worker as a coma from which the patient does not wake up.

The period of unconsciousness or coma has a wide variety of symptoms and is unpredictable. The patient needs care as well as medications but seems to be having more problems than the terminally ill. This is because the signs and symptoms are totally unpredictable, leading to deceptive conclusions. There is little or no cure at all, basically the patient is suffering continually. To clarify this the worker is faced very often with a patient who does not complain, often able to show signs of recognition, has kept almost normal body functions but in fact there is severe brain damage. Different medications have been tried with only little success. It seems to be that younger children recover more than older people however there are disabilities after recovery.

For Christian believers, what is the best way to care for these people? To my understanding the patient with persistent vegetative state is in a condition between life and death, even between heaven and hell. In the best sellers book by Dr. Maurice Rawlings, cardio vascular surgeon describes how patients in the in-between stages could see different scenes. This happens repeatedly after cardio vascular resuscitation, when patients return from death. He made sure that he interviewed them immediately after they came back to life. If he waited longer they often forget what they saw, in other words these particular patients with Persistent Vegetative Syndrome are most likely experiencing the same feelings, so how can we help them as a worker? If it is true that they change from one place to another, they need all the support we can give. What then can we give other than prayers? How can we walk with the person if we do not walk with Jesus because Jesus has the keys of hell and can determine who should go in or not.

Ref: ""BEYOND DEATH'S DOORS" by dr.Maurice Rawlings.

Reference: http://en.wikipendia.org/wiki/Persistent_vegetative_state#Definition

Dr. Francis Dartana
#219-3243 Cowichan Lake Rd
Duncan, B.C. V9L 4B8

ARMOR OF LOVE

SELF-COMPOSED SONG BY FRANCES S.H.DARTANA
To be used with the tune from "Tennessee waltz"

In His Image, in His Image,
With perfection He made me,
And gave me an armor of love!
With my feet shed with the gospel
My breastplate of righteousness,
I march to the Mansions Above!

With the girdle of truth,
The helmet of salvation,
God used them to slaughter the foe!
With the Words of the Spirit
And the large Shield of Faith then,
We proceed till the Heavens aglow!

CHAPTER X

Faith, Hope, Expectations

Hebrew's 11: 1

Faith is the substance of things hoped for

How do I understand this? It means that faith is a very important factor in the concepts of life and death. For instance if a person's hope is life, and has done everything to promote that, the substance is life and is there, already present as a reality. (For example: already a truth, an existing reality). To my understanding, the same is true for death.

Expectations of a hospice worker: I suggest keeping the main attention to the next sentence of the same verse where we read: "Faith is the evidence of things not seen"; therefore, working with faith is of the utmost importance during prayer and bedside care for anyone who is terminally ill. What about expectations? Best is to consider again the facts mentioned in the addendum . . . about the hospice and certainly at any time consider brain death, especially when the individual is relatively young and certain parts of the brain seem to be still functioning as we know, medical reassessment is helpful and can give answers.

Expectations in close relatives must be guided by counselors who are aware of emotional over involvement such as was the case with Terry Schiafo. Dr. Maurice Rawlings wrote in his book: "Beyond death's door" on several of his resuscitated patients who died then lived a very short time after that they actually could see and experience scenes of Heaven or Hell.

Now if Hell is a reality for some of us, where as it was in essence meant for the Devil and his Angels, we can see what the patient may think. With proper counseling and again positive attitude (because we may be in the DOUBT SITUATION we should try to lead the patient into more conclusive statements. And certainly there should be regular intensive soul searching where by the worker may see him/ herself as a warrior. This means he prays against all the strong holds between the patient and heaven. As we know there are many religions and we need to spend time studying. Again this is regarding Heaven and Hell.

So once again, hoping is good positive thinking and should be on each worker's agenda. No doubt that the Joy of the Lord is our strength; King David always used music to encourage his soldiers.

However, there must be a strong underlying basis of faith in the promises of God or for some of us just "a HIGHER POWER" in order to persevere when nothing happens and everything remains UNSEEN. As we know, this often happens in patients with PERSISTENT VEGETATIVE STATE. As a nurse or skilled hospice worker one must walk close to JESUS, WHO HOLDS THE KEYS OF HELL.

In several ministries the "Laying on of hands" is used, whereby the worker's hand touches softly to the pain inside, while the others pray. God can let HIS HEALING or relief stream thru the hand.

When I was about 20 years old, something similar happened which I did not understand. I was praying the "Our Father" at the bedside of an elderly lady relative who was in coma due to brain-tumor. She fell asleep and died. To me it seems like a co-incident, but imagine God willing to use your hands for many such purposes?

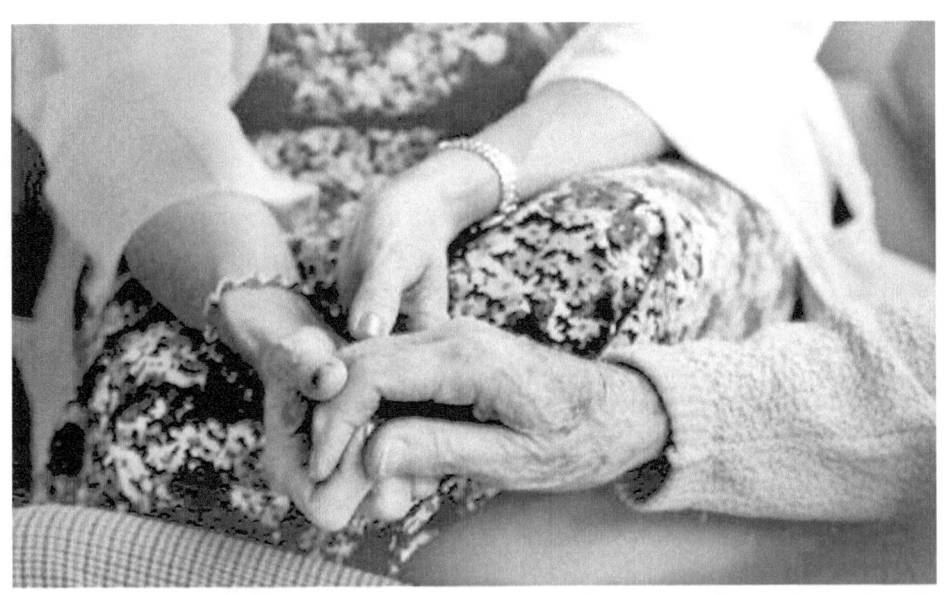

"Helping Hands"

CHAPTER XI

Funeral as a Celebration

When going thru the stages of grief: anger, denial, negotiation, 'it will be followed by acceptance meaning total liberation. I believe the same stages occur in life and terminal illness.

Acceptance and liberation: how wonderful! Comparable with a lovely song sung by two singers in one accord. Acceptance means the falling off of chains, running away or flying away in clear blue skies. We may still cry but these are tears of joy!

Such is the liberation stage for the silent grief "prison" of the terminally ill. A funeral is a temporary farewell with a reunion in sight. The only problems will be around the feelings of missing or loss of the deceased. Those may stay for long periods of time despite counseling. So in fact it is a normal happening. I think there will be many questions about being able to speak with the deceased for the other people left behind and it is the duty of the hospice worker to help them either understand or accept.

It is not hard to imagine how the angels will welcome us the redeemed people. From the song "Amazing Grace" one hears "I once was lost but now I'm found was blind but now I see. In complete silent times the worker can often go thru the various aspects of Heaven, such as the Gate of Pearl and the streets of gold. Readings about the various aspects of Heaven is one of the aggressive ways within our capacity to combat fight against sadness about life.

When we touch the lifeless body of the deceased we know that the same is now decorated and honored with a glorified body, such as Jesus carried after Resurrection

CHAPTER XII

SONGS TO ACCOMPANY

PSALM 91:

**FOR ALL OF US WHO DWELL IN SECRET PLACES OF
THE MOST HIGH SOVEREIGN GOD.
WE WILL REMAIN IN THE SHADOWS OF THE
ALMIGHTY**

WHEN ALL I HAVE IS STONES AND SLING
MY STRENGTH COMES FROM THE LORD.
FOR ALL I HAVE IS HIS TO GIVE,
MY TRUST IS IN THE LORD.

WHEN ALL MY WALLS KEEP BREAKING DOWN
MY TRUST STAYS IN THE LORD.
HE KEEPS ME UP AND GUIDES ME THROUGH
MY TRUST ENDS IN THE LORD.

NO WEAPONS FORMED AGAINST ME STAND
MY TRUST IS IN THE LORD.
NO TEAR I SHED IS WASTED YET,

MY STRENGTH IS IN THE LORD.

WHEN ALL OF US WILL SEE YOUR FACE,
WE PUT OUR TRUST IN YOU.
WE HOLD YOUR BANNER IN OUR HANDS,
AND HOLD YOUR VICTORY TOO.

WHEN ROARING LIONS WALK AROUND
TO FIND AND CAN DEVOUR
MY STRENGTH IS HIS WORD.
I SPEAK THE WORD, THE ONLY WORD,
MY STRENGTH IS IN THE LORD!

WHEN ALL I HAVE IS STONES AND SLING
MY STRENGTH COMES FROM THE LORD.
FOR ALL I HAVE IS HIS TO GIVE,
MY TRUST IS IN THE LORD.

WHEN ALL MY WALLS KEEP BREAKING DOWN
MY TRUST STAYS IN THE LORD.
HE KEEPS ME UP AND GUIDES ME THROUGH
MY TRUST ENDS IN THE LORD.

NO WEAPONS FORMED AGAINST ME STAND
MY TRUST IS IN THE LORD.
NO TEAR I SHED IS WASTED YET,
MY STRENGTH IS IN THE LORD.

WHEN ALL OF US WILL SEE YOUR FACE,
WE PUT OUR TRUST IN YOU.
WE HOLD YOUR BANNER IN OUR HANDS,
AND HOLD YOUR VICTORY TOO.

TUNE: AULD LANG SYNE

THE THORNS OF THE FLESH

IN THESE VERY DEEP DARKER VALLEYS,
GOD'S LOVE OVERFLOWS IN MY HEART!
NO WORDS CAN DESCRIBE ALL THE SORROW,
HIS GRACE IS SUFFICIENT FOR ME . . .

I DWELL IN HIS MOST SECRET PLACES,
AND DEEP IN THE PALM OF HIS HAND.
HIS LOVE AND HIS GLORY IN MY HEART
WILL SHOW HIS TRUE FACE TO THE WORLD.

MY BOTH FEET ARE SHOD WITH THE GOSPEL
AND ANGELS GUARD ME AROUND.
THE GIRDLE OF TRUTH ON MY BOTH LOINS
THE HELM OF SALVATION IS ON.

THE SWORD OF THE SPIRIT IN MY HAND
WILL WARD OFF PLANS OF THE FOE.
BY BEING A FULLY DRESSED WARRIOR,
HIS GRACE IS SUFFICIENT FOR ME

THE DOVE

COME,HOLY SPIRIT COME.
THIS IS A BRANDNEW DAY,
COME AND FILL US.

WE'RE ASKING YOU TO STAY,
AND FILL US WITH YOUR LIGHT
AND ALL YOUR LOVE.

OH GIVE US COMFORT TOO,
YOU SWEET AND GENTLE DOVE!
BLESS US AGAIN.

BRING FLOWERS FOR THE DAY
BALMS AND OINTMENTS TOO,
OH LOVELY DOVE!

THEN FILL US WITH YOUR FIRE,
POWER AND WISDOM TOO,
RESTORE OUR PEACE.

COME WITH YOUR HEALING POWER
AND TOUCH ME ONCE AGAIN,WITH BEAUTY

THEN HOVERING ABOVE,
WITH ALL YOUR JOY AND STRENGTH
UPLIFT ME NOW!

LORD LEAD US IN YOUR WAYS
YOU KNOW THE PROMISED LAND
AND PASTURES GREEN!

YOU ARE THE RISEN LORD,
THE KEYS OF HELL ARE YOURS,
FOREVER KING!

MARANATHA

So we sing Lord
You will come back
Be amongst us;
Even so Lord, come now quickly;
We are ready, We are ready!

To all Nations, came to the promise
of your coming, for deliverance!
we have seen you
recognized you,
keep the light lord,
in our eyes, lord.

you are wonderful,
ever tender, loving kindness.
maranatha, brilliant victor!
no more weeping, no more crying,
you are glory!

all religions will be gathered
when you come back, and invite all.
no more breaking, between people,
they will all sit at your table!

AMAZING GRACE

AMAZING GRACE, HOW SWEET THE SOUND
THAT SAVED A WRETCH LIKE ME
I ONCE WAS LOST BUT NOW AM FOUND
WAS BLIND BUT NOW I SEE !

'TWAS GRACE THAT TAUGHT MY HEART TO FEAR
AND GRACE MY FEARS RELIEVED
HOW PRECIOUS DID THAT GRACE APPEAR
THE HOUR I FIRST BELIEVED!

THRO MANY DANGERS TOILS AND SNARES,
I HAVE ALREADY COME
THIS GRACE HAS BROUGHT ME SAFE THUS FAR
AND GRACE WILL LEAD ME HOME.

WHEN WE'VE BEEN THERE TEN THOUSAND YEARS
BRIGHT SHINING AS THE SUN
WE'VE NO LESS DAYS TO SING GOD'S PRAISE
THAN WHEN WE FIRST BEGUN.

5.PRAISE GOD.

6.LORD GOD.

7. SERVE GOD.

8. LOVE GOD.

9. THANK GOD.

Correspondence with the President and the executive director of association for the prevention of euthanasia. (Translation from Dutch)

Box 25033
London, Ont.
N6C6A8

Dear Dr. Veder & Mr. Alex Schadenberg

I have received your name from Dr. C. Persaud and I am very pleased to find friends who are willing to fight against the continuation of euthanasia and with me to fight against the bad policy. In fact it is that I encounter amazing situations where as the victims already protected still had to undergo death against their will.

The reason that I write this is that I have written a book a few years ago with the title "Complete Passionate care instead of Euthanasia". In this book I described certain ways to approach the patient psychologically, this is one of the ways to decrease pain and suffering. As you know we Doctors have been looking for medications that will decrease pain, and which are effective. There are no good reason anymore for euthanasia, that's why many people use the argument of life being worthless in certain circumstances like depression. In your letter you wrote that you also are working on a book with similar topic; of course there will be more explanations. I would like to send my book to you, perhaps you could combine the two of them? I have not published my book I hope to hear from you soon.

Friendly greetings
S.H. Dartana

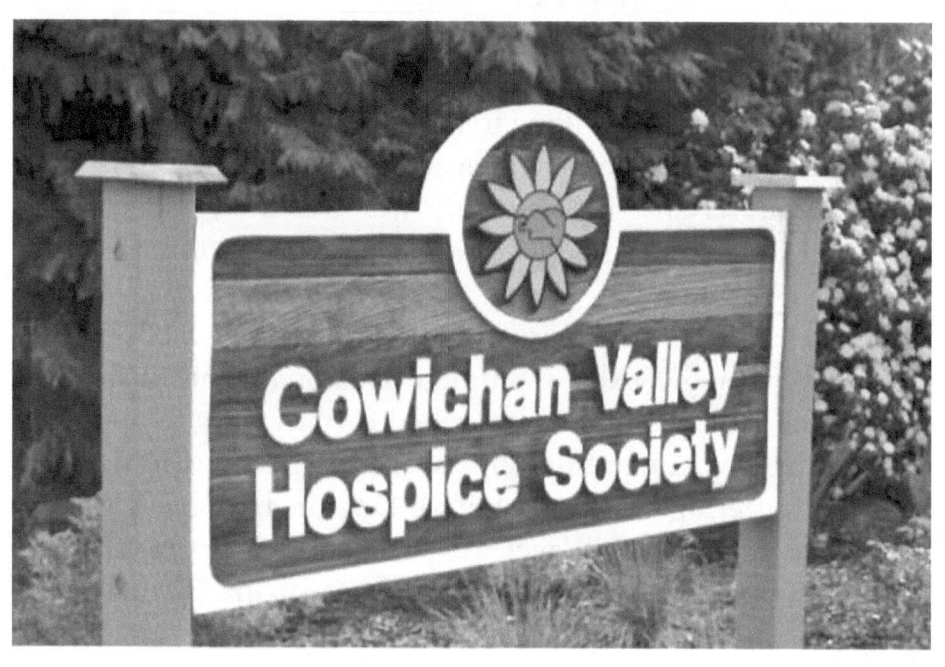

Euthanasia Prevention Coalition Newsletter
—December 2008

Landscape Evolves for assisted suicide
By Alex Schadenberg

An article by Jane Gross in the *New York Times* (November 10) examines the landscape or the changes in relation to the issue of assisted suicide since 1991 when Dr. Timothy Quill published an account of his role in the death of one of his patients.

The article makes some points that need to be examined further if we are to respond effectively to future initiatives to legalize assisted suicide.

The article describes the conditions for assisted suicide in Oregon and Washington:

> "State residents requesting this assistance must be mentally competent, have six months or less to live according to two physicians, wait 15 days after their request and then repeat that request orally and in writing. They must be capable of administering medication themselves and agree to counseling if their physicians request it. The patients also must be told of alternatives."

Dr. Quill, who is the director of the palliative care program at the University of Rochester, is quoted as saying, "these options have gained acceptance over the past decade."

The article comments on the 1997 Supreme Court ruling, as follows:

> "there was no constitutional right to physician-assisted suicide and upheld a prohibition against it. But in the ruling, the justices conceded that terminally ill

patients were entitled to aggressive pain management,
even if opiates or barbiturates had the 'double effect'
of hastening death."

The statement concerning the "double effect" principle is
inappropriately worded because the use of opiates or barbiturates
for the aggressive management of pain when it is not intended to
cause death, and therefore when properly administered, should
not be associated with assisted suicide.

A physician should not consider the "double effect" principle
as an open window to euthanasia because that is an abuse of its
proper use.

The article quotes Quill concerning the options that should
exist before one considers what he would call the "last resort" of
assisted suicide:

> "all terminally ill patients should have access to
> palliative care, both to relieve pain and other symptoms
> and to provide emotional support to patients and
> families."

But it must be stated that when palliative care is not accessible
for all people needing pain and symptom management, then
assisted suicide is an abuse of the vulnerable person who is actually
seeking relief from their suffering, not assisted suicide.

Quill recommends that a palliative care consultation be
mandatory before anyone considers a "last resort" measure. Quill
suggests that other options be made known to the patient, such
as:

- Pain management so aggressive that it may well hasten
  death, although that is not the primary intention. (This
  is the doctrine of "double effect.")

- Invoking a patient's right to forgo life-sustaining therapies or discontinue them.
- Voluntarily stopping eating and drinking. (Dr. Quill believes this is a "more morally complex" choice because over the last decade the practice has expanded beyond those with end-stage cancer or Alzheimer's disease who often lose interest in food or forget how to eat and drink to people who are not "actively dying" but nevertheless have had enough of disability or dependence).
- Sedation to the point of unconsciousness. (Although it was endorsed this year by a panel of the American Medical Association, Dr. Quill called it the "last, last resort.")"

Quill does not acknowledge that people who voluntarily stop eating or drinking when they are not "actively dying" are often people who are suffering from undiagnosed clinical depression. Physicians should uphold a pledge that they will "do no harm" which should include protecting the vulnerable.

The primary concern around the sedation of a person to the point of unconsciousness is that usually sedation includes the intentional dehydration of the person. It is sometimes necessary to sedate a person to the point of unconsciousness in order to relieve their neuropathic pain, but to intentionally dehydrate a person, who is not otherwise dying, is euthanasia by dehydration.

The article is correct when it states that the landscape has changed in relation to assisted suicide. What has not changed is the effect assisted suicide has on the attitude and treatment that is offered to people at the most vulnerable time of their life.

The question whether we need to strive for a culture that solves its difficult human problems by caring for the patient or a culure that solves its most difficult human problems by killing the patient?

I choose to care.

Euthanasia Prevention Coalition Newsletter— December 2008

Italian Court approves death by dehydration for Eluana Englaro

Italian politicians, Catholic leaders and the family of Terri Schiavo have condemned the court decision to allow the feeding tube to be removed from Eluana Englaro, which would cause her to die by dehydration.

The judges rejected the appeal of a lower court ruling in Milan resulting in Eluana's father being granted permission to have his daughter's fluids and food removed.

Cardinal Baragan, head of the Pontifical Council for Health stated, "to suspend hydration and nutrition in a patient in a vegetative state worsens his or her condition and leads to a terrible death by hunger and thirst."

The position of the Euthanasia Prevention Coalition is that removing fluids and food from Eluana Englaro is euthanasia by dehydration, because Englaro would die from intentional dehydration and not from a medical condition. Just because Englaro is cognitively disabled doesn't mean that she is not human and deserving of death by dehydration.

The Terri Schindler Schiavo Foundation stated in a press release:

> "Italy's top appeals court upheld a July ruling allowing a father to remove basic care—food and water—from his 35-year-old daughter.
>
> "Eluana Englaro has been receiving food and water via a feeding tubesince a 1992 car crash that left her with a brain injury. Her father, Beppino Englaro, has been seeking to end her life for nearly 10 years. Today's ruling will clear the way for Eluana to experience a barbaric and inhumane death by starvation and dehydration."

Bobby Schindler stated in July 2008 that

> "This court's ruling seems to indicate that American 'medical ethics' are spreading like a virus among the international community, threatening countless numbers of elderly, ailing and disabled persons in an increasing and alarming way."

> "Our heart goes out to this family as we know very well the profound effect that these types of injuries can have on loved ones. However, we must remember that we have a grave obligation to do all we can to protect those with disabilities, recognizing that a person with a brain injury is a human being with an inherent dignity and a right to life. This young girl needs only food and water and her family's love to survive. At the very least this should be provided to her."

At the time of publication of this newsletter, it is reported that the nuns who run the hospice in which Eluana has been living for 14 years have refused to carry out the court order to remove her food and hydration tube. In a letter published in *Avvenire*, the daily newspaper of the Italian Bishops Conference, the Misericordine nuns of Lecco said, "Our hope, and that of many like us, is that the death by hunger and thirst of Eluana, and others in her condition, will not be carried out."

Washington DC Hospital Sues to Remove 12-year-old Boy from Life Support

With many similarities to the Winnipeg case of Samuel Golubchuk, the Children's National Medical Center has initiated a legal battle with the family of a 12-year-old boy to discontinue life support.

Eluzer & Miriam Brody, the parents of 12-year-old Mot Brody, are trying to prevent the hospital from taking their son off life support.

The Brody family who are orthodox Jews, have retained a lawyer stated that the boy's circulatory and respiratory systems are functioning, even though they require mechanical assistance.

The hospital stated in their filing to the D.C., Supreme Court that: they extend their sympathy to the family but "scarce resources are being used for the preservation of a deceased body."

Jeffery Zucherman, the lawyer for the Brody family stated: "Under Jewish law and their faith, there is no such thing as brain death and their religious beliefs are entitled to respect."

Sophia Smith, one of the boy's physicians wrote in court papers, "This child ceased to exist be every medical definition." She added that the staff members are: "distraught at what is providing futile care to the earthly remains of a former life."

Zucherman stated that he is challenging the hospital's plans on grounds that the family's religious beliefs must be respected under federal law. He said.

George Annas, a law professor at Boston University who specializes in health law and bioethics stated, "The case law is clear: once you are dead, you are dead."

Annas added that New York and New Jersey have provisions in law that make exceptions in similar instances for Orthodox Jews but DC does not.

The Euthanasia Prevention Coalition recognizes that these are very difficult cases. Someone who is actually dead should be treated with dignity, but 'let go'. But we must always give the benefit of the doubt, especially when futile care rules are used to pressure families to prematurely stop medical care often based on cost containment principles and 'Peter singer' ethics.

Euthanasia Prevention Coalition Newsletter— December 2008

"I-1000" passes in Washington State making it the second state to legalize assisted suicide
By: Alex Schadenberg

Voters in Washington State have passed "I-1000"," thereby legalizing "Oregon style" assisted suicide by 81 to 19 percent and moderates supported assisted suicide by 63 to 37 percent.

Voters who identified themselves as Chritian, either Protestant or Catholic, were divided 50-50 on the necessity of legal protection for the vulnerable in our society.

Opponents of assisted suicide realize how grave a decision Washington State voters have made.

Assisted suicide directly threatens the lives of the most vulnerable people in our culture—people with disabilities the dependent elderly, those who live with depression and mental illness and others. It is they who will be directly threatened by assisted suicide in Washington State.

People who believe that I-1000 will not lead to a slippery slope should read the comments by Ted Goodwin, President of the Final Exit Network, in a press release on November 5, 2008:

Although the supporters of I-1000 are delighted that Washington becomes the second state to pass a "Death with Dignity Act", there is much more to be done.

We congratulate all those who worked so hard to achieve this important right for Washington's citizens, and we applaud the citizens of Washington State for making the right choice. Final Exit Network and its members supported passage of this landmark initiatively by donating work pledges, until laws protect the right of every adult to a peaceful, dignified death, Final Exit Network will be there to support those who need relief from their suffering today!

The Network's Exit Guide Program is available nationwide, with the Network's compassionate guidance and support, physically and mentally competent adults in all fifty states are free to exercise their last human right—the right to a peaceful, dignified death. Final Exit Network is the only organization in the United States that will support individuals who are not "terminally ill"—6 months or less to live—to hasten their deaths. No other organization in the U.S. makes this commitment.

Goodwin is saying that their goal is to eliminate all barriers to euthanasia and assisted suicide.

He is also saying that they will continue to subvert the laws in the other 48 states in the U.S. as well as offer assisted suicide to people who do not qualify for legal assisted suicide in Oregon and Washington.

Goodwin and other leaders in the euthanasia lobby will continue to push for changes until they have achieved the final goal—"death on demand."

The Final Exit ideology appears different from, but is actually similar to that of the Compassion & Choices lobby group who led the I-1000 assisted suicide initiative.

Compassion & Choices, the leading euthanasia lobby group, focus on spreading assisted suicide in an incremental fashion. Compassion & Choices will focus on the next State initiatives to legalize assisted suicide. Those initiatives may include another ballot initiative or they may first attempt another legislative proposal.

Once Compassion & Choices succeeds in having assisted suicide legalized in many states, they will then focus on expanding its application through legislative changes to existing statutes or through the courts.

Wesley Smith commented on the lack of financial support received by the Coalition Against Assisted Suicide compared to the Right to Die lobby.

Meanwhile, the opposition to assisted suicide is generally starved for funds, marginalized in the popular media, and as a consequence, always stuck in reactive mode when we need to be proactive.

But we can't do it alone. If people and foundations wish to stop this juggernaut, they are going to have to do what proponents have done and step forward and give those of us willing to give our all to fighting the death culture the resources we need to compete. If they don't, there will be more Washington States.

Anyone who still says "it can't happen here," isn't paying attention. It is happening here, and it will happen here increasingly unless there is greater commitment shown by those with means who oppose these agendas to reversing the current course.

Link to Weley's Smith's blog at: www.wesleyjsmith.com

For further analysis of the Washington State I-1000 assisted suicide Initiative go to International Task Force on Euthanasia and Assisted Suicide *www.internationaltaskforce.org*

The Euthanasia Prevention Coalition will continue to build a unified and organized effort of groups and individuals who are working to create a cultural barrier to euthanasia and assisted suicide while stemming the tide of the euthanasia lobby.

It is very difficult to organize and unify our efforts when we lack the necessary funds to build a stronger and more inclusive infrastructure.

Smith is correct. You will need to decide whether you are willing to invest in our work. Your support will enable us to build an effective opposition to the juggernaut of the euthanasia lobby.

It is your decision.

We know that the euthanasia lobby will continue to push their radical agenda until the right to die, becomes a duty to die.

Society needs to focus on Caring solutions to end-of-life concerns and reject killing.

To join or support the Euthanasia Prevention Coalition, contact us. Our website is at *www.epcc.ca*; e-mail: *info@epcc.ca*; call toll free: 1-888-439-3348.

Second International symposium on Euthanasia and Assisted Suicide

Plan to attend the Second International symposium on Euthanasia and Assisted Suicide entitled "Never Again" at the National Conference Center (close to Dulles International Airport and Washington DC). Cosponsors are the Euthanasia Prevention Coalition, Physicians for Compassionate Care, Not Dead Yet, the Care Not Killing Alliance and No Less Human in the UK.

This event will follow on the success of the First International Symposium, held in Toronto, which featured almost every leader on the issues of euthanasia and assisted suicide.

We have already received commitments from leading speakers in the UK, te Netherlands, Belgium, the U.S.A. and Canada.

This will be the most important conference held to date on euthanasia and assited suicide. You will leave with important information about the current issues and a clear understanding of how we are proceeding.

Euthanasia
Prevention
Coalition

November 18, 2008

Dear Friends

These are difficult times. The Euthanasia Prevention Coalition (EPC) is experiencing a financial crisis. Whether it is due to the recession or not, we are experiencing a significant shortfall in major donations.

The I-1000 assisted suicide Initiative passed making Washington State the second state to legalize assisted suicide. We are working with other leaders to analyze the results in order to stop future attempts to legalize assisted suicide. We will be organizing and preparing for the expected barrage from the euthanasia lobby in Canada, the United States and world-wide. This is the reason why we are organizing the Second International Symposium on Euthanasia and Assisted Suicide for Washington DC—May 29-30, 2009. Please plan to attend.

EPC sent a representative to the World Federation of Right to Die Societies Conference held in Paris, France October 29-November 1, 2008. It is important to know the goals and directions of the euthanasia lobby. A report of the World Federation of Right to Die Societies Conference will be available from EPC in January 2009.

The Bloc Québeçois MP Francine Lalonde (La Pointe-de-I'lle) was one of the speakers at the World Federation of Right to Die Societies Conference. She announced that she will re-introduce her private members bill to legalize euthanasia and assisted suicide in Canada. We expect that Lalonde's bill will be similar to Bill C-562 that she introduced before the last election.

Lalonde referred to the fact that there have been several cases of assisted suicide in Quebec in the past few years. She alluded to the possibility of a future case being exploited to challenge our laws through the courts.

The Euthanasia Prevention Coalition held its National Symposium in Winnipeg, October 24-25, 2008. We are fortunate to be working with the Council of Canadians with Disabilities and the Manitoba League of Persons with Disabilities. The theme for the Symposium was "Death Making".

The speakers at the Symposium followed a common theme enabling the participants to learn information and gain an understanding of the disability perspective and how it relates to end-of-life issues. All presentations were recorded and a DVD set from the Symposium will be available in January 2009. We are offering a special pre-order rate of $25.00 for the complete Symposium set.

Our donations are significantly down this year and large donations have nearly disappeared.

The reality is that *my credit card* is at its limit because I had use it to pay expenses for EPC. This is very distressing for me and my family. I have always put everything into this work but now I really need your help.

I would like to thank you for your support and hope that you can help us through these difficult times.

Alex Schadenberg
Executive Director

BIBLIOGRAPHY

42—M.R.J. ADDISON: "Concerns about the new Alberta personal directives act" Health Ethics today vol. 9, no. 1 Nov. 97 pg. 7

20—I.R. BYOCK: "Consciously Walking the Fine line: Thoughts on a Hospice; Response to Assisted Suicide and Euthanasia" Journal of Palliative care, vol. 9, 3, Autumn 1993, pp 25-28.

35—J. COULEHAN: "The man with stars inside", Annals of Internal Medicine 126[10] 788-8021997, May 15.

7—H.M. CHOCHINOV "Treating Depression in the terminally ill", Pain Management Newsletter, vol. 8 no. 1 April 1995, pp. 4-5

31—H.M. CHOCHINOV: "Desire for death in terminally ill" Pain Management Newsletter, vol. 9, no. 3, 1996, pg. 10.

6—H.M. CHOCHINOV: "Psychiatric care of the cancer patient" Medicine, North America, Nov/dec 1994, pp 671-674

32—L. COHEN: "Jewish and secular medical ethics share themes but diverge such as heroic measures." CMAJ 2997, 157, 1415-6.

42—L.M. COHEN et al.: "Dialysis discontinuation; a good death?" Arch. Intern. Medicine 1995 Jan, 155:1, 42-7.

1—C.R.S. DAWES: Letter to the Editor: "Not all Doctors Oppose Euthanasia" Canadian Medical News, May 1995, pg 2.

8—M.L. FARNCOMBE: "Nebulized Morphine" Pain Management Newsletter, vol 8, no 1 April 1995 pg 5.

37—E.A. FREEMAN: "The Coma Exit chart: assessing the patient in prolonged coma and the vegetative state" Brain Injury 10[8]: 615-24, 1996, Aug

42—A.M. FRASER: "Morrison case dismissed" The Halifax Herald, Ltd. Feb. 28, 1998.

3—S.S. GULA: "What are they saying about Euthanasia?" New York, Paulist Press, 1986.

30—H. HAYES: "Tolerance and toxicity to Opioids" Pain Management Newsletter vol 8 no 1, April 1995 pg. 8.

33—R. HEYDEMANN: "A spiritual perspective of personal directives" Health Ethics Today vol. 9 no 1, Nov 97, pg. 5.

44—T.A. HUTCHINSON et al.: "Death. A rewarding experience?" CMAJ 1997; 157: 1687-8.

9—J.M. JONES: "Review re, Continuous Subcutaneous Infusion of Analgesics" Pain Management Newsletter, vol, 8, no 1, April 1995 pg 9.

21—Senator KEON, Special Committee for Euthanasia, Teleconference in Ottawa, summer 1995.

34—W.A. LAFRANCE: "Is it ethical to forgo treatment?" CMAJ, Dec. 97; 157[12]pg 1740-41.

36—E. LATIMER: "Palliative care, easing the pain" Canadian Journal of Diagnosis, Sept. 1996, pg 97-102

29—E.J. LATIMER: "Caring for the Dying in Canada" Canadian Family Physician, vol 41 March 1995, pp362-365.

37—P.S. LINKS: "Suicide and life; the ultimate juxtaposition" JAMA 1998, 158 [4] pg. 514-515.

19—C.S.L. LIBRACH: "Special Issues in Pain Control during terminal illness", Canadian Family Physician, vol. 41, March 1995, pp. 1-3.

2—N. MACDONALD: "Interview re: Aspects of Palliative care". Pain management Newsletter, vol, 8, no, 1 April 1995, pp 1-3

38—A. MERRIMAN, C. LAN-TING: "Reactions to death and dying by doctors, medical students and nurses in Singapore

1985-1986" Annals of the Academy of Medicine, Singapore 16[1]: 133-6, 1987. Jan.

15—B. MOUNT: "Counselling as Death Approaches" Canadian Medical Association Journal, Nov. 1995, 153[9] pp. 1340-1342

18—N. NAZERALI: "Counselling the Elderly on Decision Making for the end of life" Canadian Family Physician, vol. 41, May 1995, pp. 829-833.

43—CMA POLICYBASE: "Advance directives for resuscitation and other life-saving or sustaining measures" CMAJ 1992, 146, 1072A

5—M. PICKUP: "Letters to the Editor" Journal Society of Obstetrics and Gynecology Canada. March 1995, pp. 229-230.

11—N.A SANTIN: "One Medical Student's Experience" Pain Management Newsletter, vol. 8 no, 1, April 1995, pp 2-3

25—J.F. SCOTT: "Palliative care Does not and Should not Hasten Death" Pain Management Digest and Dialogue. vol. 7, no. 4, Winter 1991, pp. 2-7.

12—P. SINGER: "Living Wills" Alberta Heritage foundation for Medical Research Newsletter, May/June 1995, pp. 9-10.

41—Rev. L. SUMRALL: "Spirit, Soul and Body" Springdale, Pennsylvania, Whittaker House, 1995.

4—Rev. G. TATTRIE: "Euthanasia, a Christian Perspective" Don Mills, Board of Congregational Life. the Presbyterian Church in Canada, 1982.

39—Y. QUEENEVILLE: "Facing the emotional pain of others" Pain Management Newsletter vol. 19, 1996, pg, 12.

40—K.G. WILSON et al: "Talking to the terminally ill about euthanasia and physician assisted suicide" Can. J. of Clinical medicine, vol. 5 no. 4, pg. 68-74, April 1998

www.ingramcontent.com/pod-product-compliance
Lightning Source LLC
Chambersburg PA
CBHW021240280526
45784CB00005B/2170